Homemade Body Butter

25 Natural, Preservative-Free Recipes for Homemade Body Butter

Table of Contents

Introduction

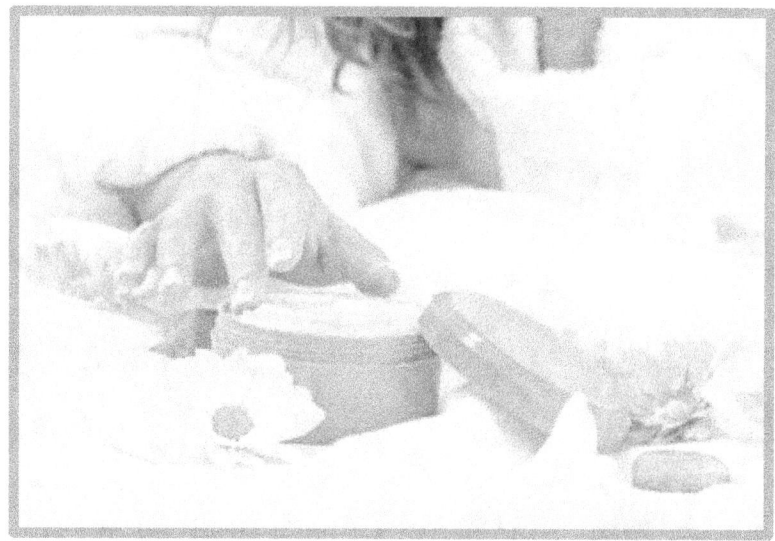

If you go to a bath and body shop or a spa boutique, you will find an assortment of lotions, creams and ointments for every skin ailment or condition you can think of. What you may not realize, however, is that you do not need to buy a different product for all of your skin woes – there is one product that has a number of different uses – body butter. Body butter is a thick moisturizing cream that can be used to moisturize your skin, to smooth rough patches, to soften cuticles and as a lip balm. You can even use body butter to soothe your skin after shaving and to remove eye make-up! This product is one that every woman should have in her arsenal.

Given the multifunctional nature of body butter, you may think that you have to spend a lot of money for a good one. The reality is, however, that you can make your very own body butter at home! In this book you will find a collection of 25 different recipes for creating homemade body butter. These body butter recipes will yield luxurious, moisturizing body butter than can be used on your hands, feet, face and skin. After reading this book you may never purchase body butter from a bath and beauty shop again!

Homemade Body Butter Recipes

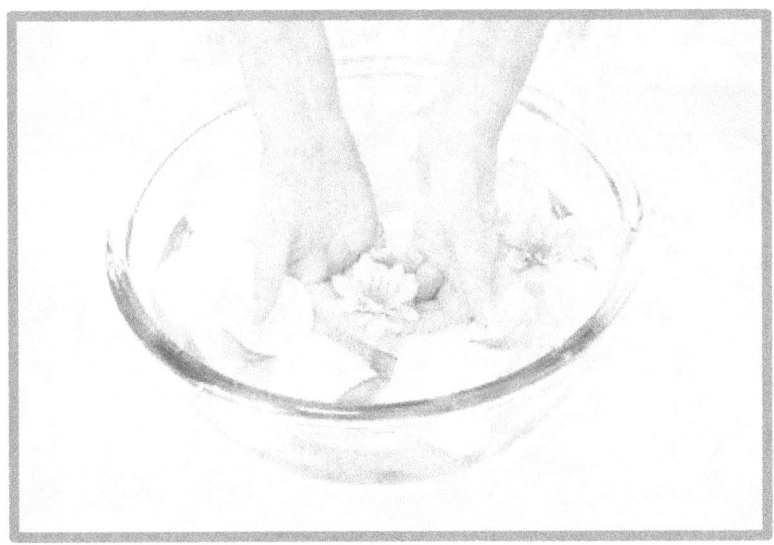

Recipes Included in this Book:

Basic Body Butter

Shea Body Butter

Vanilla Body Butter

Whipped Lavender Body Butter

Peppermint Body Butter

Antibacterial Body Butter

Sweet Citrus Body Butter

Coconut Oil Body Butter

Aromatherapy Body Butter

Rosemary Tallow Body Butter

Cocoa Cinnamon Body Butter

Olive Oil Body Butter

Vitamin E Body Butter

Mango Body Butter

Soothing Coconut Oil Body Butter

Sandalwood Body Butter

Relaxing Bergamot Body Butter

Chamomile Body Butter

Sweet Cedarwood Body Butter

Bug Repellant Body Butter

Mood-Lifting Body Butter

Fresh and Floral Body Butter

Astringent Body Butter

Jasmine Body Butter

Basic Body Butter

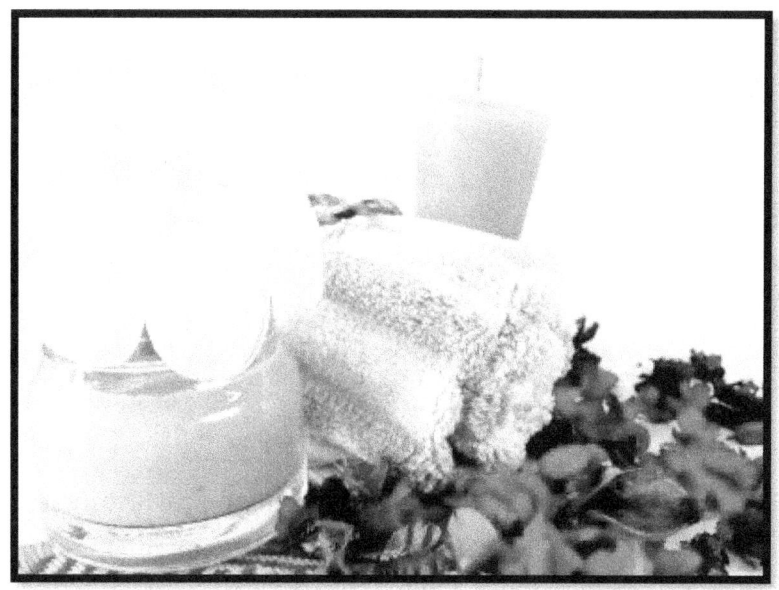

Ingredients:

½ cup coconut oil

1/3 cup cocoa butter

2 tablespoons sweet almond oil

Scant ¼ teaspoon tea tree oil

Instructions:

1. Heat the cocoa butter in a double boiler over low heat until just melted.
2. Remove from heat and whisk in the coconut oil and sweet almond oil.
3. Let the mixture solidify at room temperature.
4. Whip the body butter on high speed for 5 to 8 minutes, scraping down the sides as needed.
5. Add the tea tree oil then beat again.
6. Transfer the body butter to a glass or plastic jar and seal it with a lid.

Vanilla Body Butter

Ingredients:

1 cup cocoa butter

½ cup coconut oil

1/3 cup sweet almond oil

1 dried vanilla bean

Instructions:

1. Heat the cocoa butter in a double boiler over low heat until just melted.
2. Remove from heat and whisk in the coconut oil and sweet almond oil.
3. Grind the vanilla bean in a coffee grinder and stir into the oil.
4. Let the mixture solidify at room temperature.
5. Whip the body butter on high speed for 5 to 8 minutes, scraping down the sides as needed.
6. Transfer the body butter to a glass or plastic jar and seal it with a lid.

Whipped Lavender Body Butter

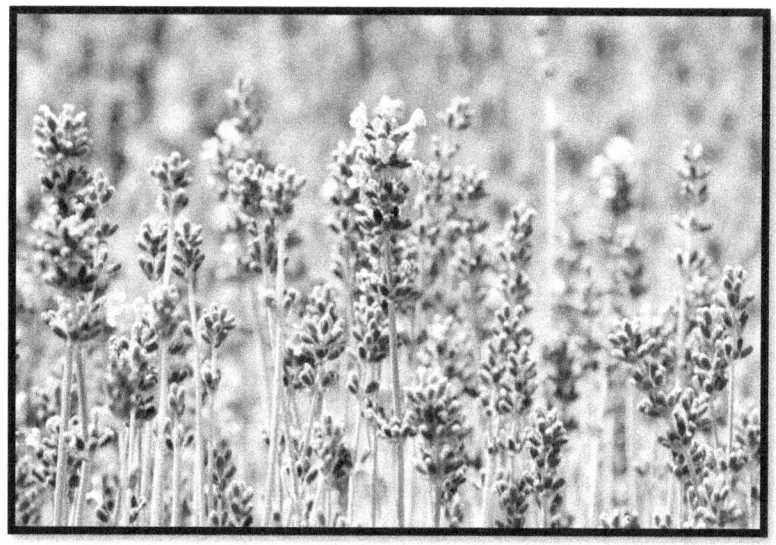

Ingredients:

½ cup coconut oil

1/3 cup cocoa butter

2 tablespoons jojoba oil

10 drops lavender essential oil

5 drops tea tree oil

Instructions:

1. Heat the cocoa butter in a double boiler over low heat until just melted.
2. Remove from heat and whisk in the coconut oil and sweet almond oil.
3. Let the mixture solidify at room temperature.
4. Whip the body butter on high speed for 5 to 8 minutes, scraping down the sides as needed.
5. Add the tea tree oil then beat again.
6. Transfer the body butter to a glass or plastic jar and seal it with a lid.

Shea Body Butter

Ingredients:

1 cup shea butter

½ cup coconut oil

½ cup jojoba oil

10 to 20 drops essential oil (you may combine oils)

Instructions:

1. Heat the shea butter in a double boiler over low heat until just melted.
2. Remove from heat and whisk in the coconut oil and jojoba oil.
3. Let the mixture solidify at room temperature.
4. Whip the body butter on high speed for 5 to 8 minutes, scraping down the sides as needed.
5. Add the essential oil then beat again.
6. Transfer the body butter to a glass or plastic jar and seal it with a lid.

Sweet Citrus Body Butter

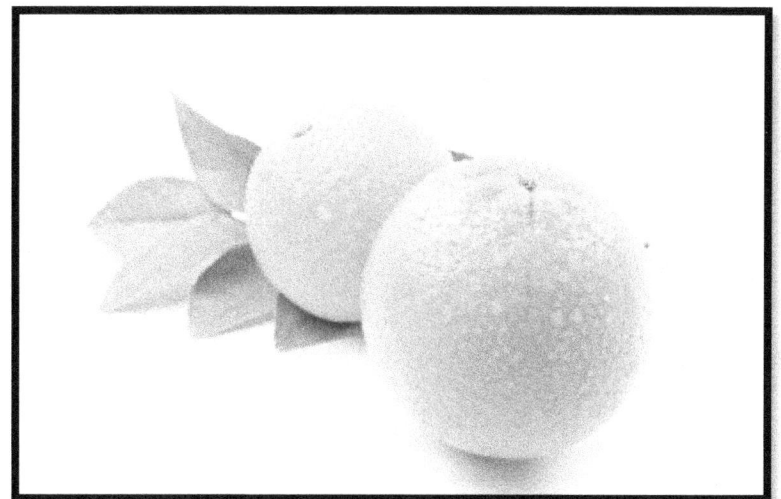

Ingredients:

½ cup cocoa butter

½ cup mango butter

½ cup coconut oil

½ cup sweet almond oil

10 drops orange essential oil

5 drops lemon essential oil

Instructions:

1. Heat the cocoa butter and mango butter in a double boiler over low heat until just melted.
2. Remove from heat and whisk in the coconut oil and sweet almond oil.
3. Let the mixture solidify at room temperature.
4. Whip the body butter on high speed for 5 to 8 minutes.
5. Add the essential oils then beat again.
6. Transfer the body butter to a glass or plastic jar and seal it with a lid.

Peppermint Body Butter

Ingredients:

½ cup cocoa butter

½ cup coconut oil

½ cup shea butter

½ cup jojoba oil

3 drops peppermint essential oil

Instructions:

1. Heat the cocoa butter in a double boiler over low heat until just melted.
2. Remove from heat and whisk in the coconut oil, shea butter and jojoba oil.
3. Let the mixture solidify at room temperature.
4. Whip the body butter on high speed for 5 to 8 minutes, scraping down the sides as needed.
5. Add the peppermint oil then beat again.
6. Transfer the body butter to a glass or plastic jar and seal it with a lid.

Coconut Oil Body Butter

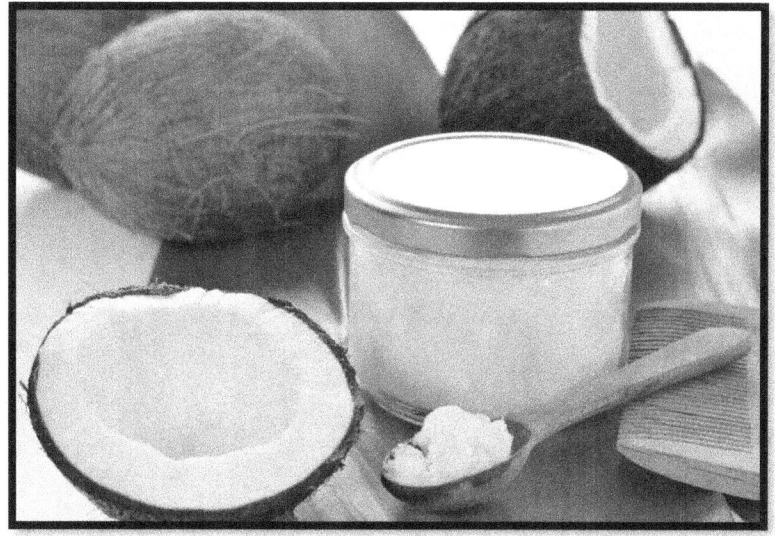

Ingredients:

1 cup coconut oil

1 teaspoon sweet almond oil

2 to 3 drops essential oil (try rose, lemon or citron)

Instructions:

1. Combine the coconut oil, sweet almond oil and essential oil in a mixing bowl.
2. Whip the body butter on high speed for 5 to 8 minutes, scraping down the sides as needed.
3. Transfer the body butter to a glass or plastic jar and seal it with a lid.

Antibacterial Body Butter

Ingredients:

½ cup shea butter

¼ cup coconut oil

¼ cup jojoba oil

5 drops eucalyptus essential oil

5 drops tea tree oil

1 to 2 drops fragrant essential oil (rosemary, lavender, orange)

Instructions:

1. Heat the shea butter in a double boiler over low heat until just melted.
2. Remove from heat and whisk in the coconut oil and jojoba oil.
3. Let the mixture solidify at room temperature.
4. Whip the body butter on high speed for 5 to 8 minutes, scraping down the sides as needed.
5. Add the eucalyptus oil, tea tree oil and fragrant oil then beat again.
6. Transfer the body butter to a glass or plastic jar and seal it with a lid.

Cocoa Cinnamon Body Butter

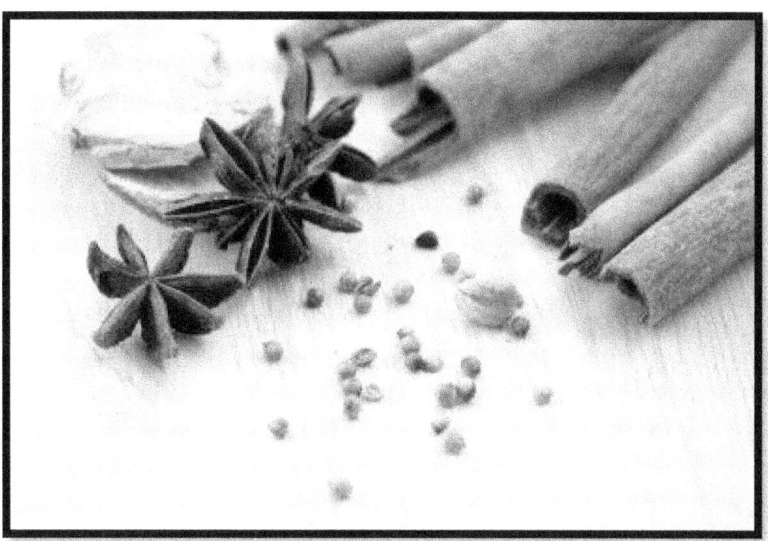

Ingredients:

1 cup cocoa butter

½ cup coconut oil

¼ cup sweet almond oil

1 tablespoon jojoba oil

3 to 5 drops cinnamon essential oil

Instructions:

1. Heat the cocoa butter in a double boiler over low heat until just melted.
2. Remove from heat and whisk in the coconut oil, jojoba and sweet almond oil.
3. Let the mixture solidify at room temperature.
4. Whip the body butter on high speed for 5 to 8 minutes, scraping down the sides as needed.
5. Add the cinnamon essential oil then beat again.
6. Transfer the body butter to a glass or plastic jar and seal it with a lid.

Aromatherapy Body Butter

Ingredients:

½ cup coconut oil

1/3 cup cocoa butter

2 tablespoons jojoba oil

5 drops jasmine essential oil

5 drops rosewood essential oil

Instructions:

1. Heat the cocoa butter in a double boiler over low heat until just melted.
2. Remove from heat and whisk in the coconut oil and jojoba oil.
3. Let the mixture solidify at room temperature.
4. Whip the body butter on high speed for 5 to 8 minutes, scraping down the sides as needed.
5. Add the essential oils then beat again.
6. Transfer the body butter to a glass or plastic jar and seal it with a lid.

Olive Oil Body Butter

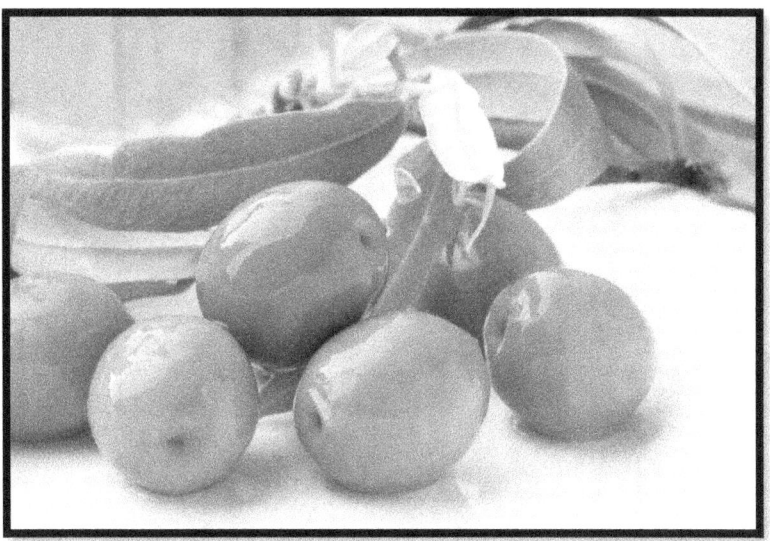

Ingredients:

1 cup cocoa butter

½ cup coconut oil

½ cup light olive oil

10 to 15 drops essential oil (optional)

Instructions:

1. Heat the cocoa butter in a double boiler over low heat until just melted.
2. Remove from heat and whisk in the coconut oil and olive oil.
3. Let the mixture solidify at room temperature.
4. Whip the body butter on high speed for 5 to 8 minutes, scraping down the sides as needed.
5. Add the essential oils, if using, then beat again.
6. Transfer the body butter to a glass or plastic jar and seal it with a lid.

Rosemary Tallow Body Butter

Ingredients:

1 cup shea butter

½ cup tallow

1/3 cup jojoba oil

2 tablespoons sweet almond oil

1 teaspoon rosemary essential oil

Instructions:

1. Heat the shea butter and tallow in a double boiler over low heat until just melted.
2. Remove from heat and whisk in the jojoba oil and sweet almond oil.
3. Let the mixture solidify at room temperature.
4. Whip the body butter on high speed for 5 to 8 minutes, scraping down the sides as needed.
5. Add the rosemary oil then beat again.
6. Transfer the body butter to a glass or plastic jar and seal it with a lid.

Mango Body Butter

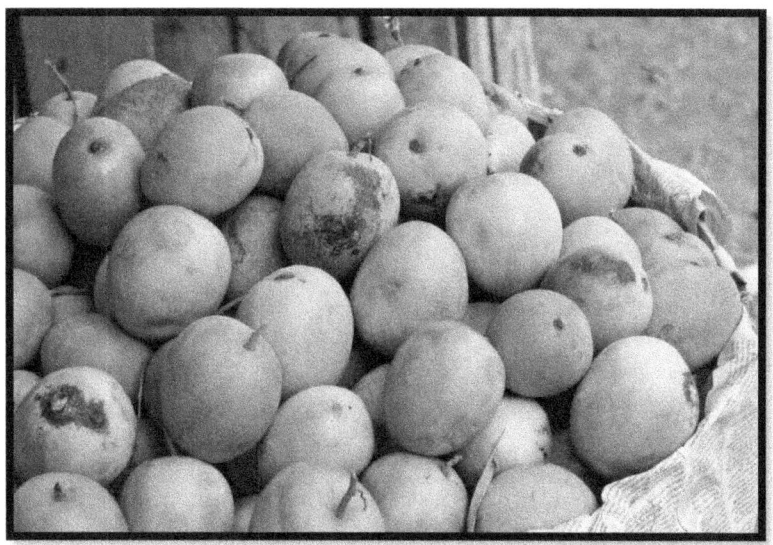

Ingredients:

½ cup mango butter

½ cup shea butter

½ cup coconut oil

½ cup jojoba oil

10 to 15 drops citrus essential oil

Instructions:

1. Heat the mango butter and shea butter in a double boiler over low heat until just melted.
2. Remove from heat and whisk in the coconut oil and jojoba oil.
3. Let the mixture solidify at room temperature.
4. Whip the body butter on high speed for 5 to 8 minutes, scraping down the sides as needed.
5. Add the citrus essential oil then beat again.
6. Transfer the body butter to a glass or plastic jar and seal it with a lid.

Vitamin E Body Butter

Ingredients:

½ cup coconut oil

1/3 cup cocoa butter

2 tablespoons sweet almond oil

1 teaspoon vitamin E oil

5 to 10 drops essential oil

Instructions:

1. Heat the cocoa butter in a double boiler over low heat until just melted.
2. Remove from heat and whisk in the coconut oil and sweet almond oil.
3. Let the mixture solidify at room temperature.
4. Whip the body butter on high speed for 5 to 8 minutes, scraping down the sides as needed.
5. Add the vitamin E oil and essential oil then beat again.
6. Transfer the body butter to a glass or plastic jar and seal it with a lid.

Relaxing Bergamot Body Butter

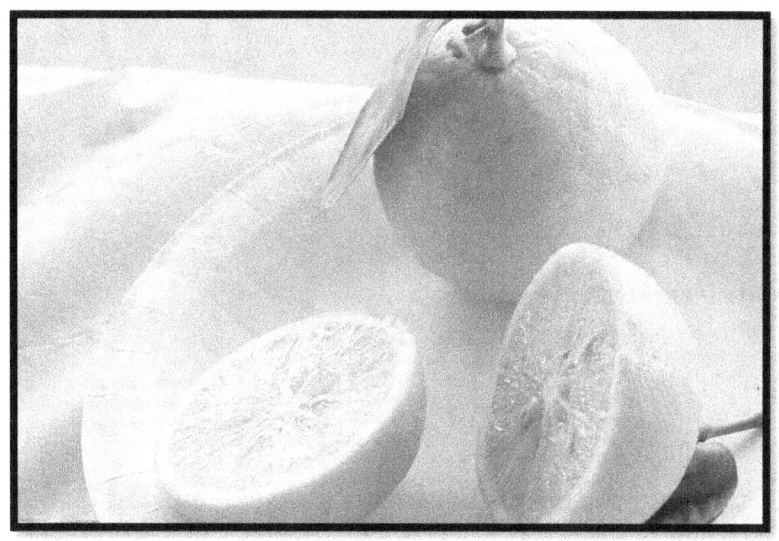

Ingredients:

½ cup coconut oil

1/3 cup cocoa butter

2 tablespoons jojoba oil

10 drops bergamot essential oil

Instructions:

1. Heat the cocoa butter in a double boiler over low heat until just melted.
2. Remove from heat and whisk in the coconut oil and jojoba oil.
3. Let the mixture solidify at room temperature.
4. Whip the body butter on high speed for 5 to 8 minutes, scraping down the sides as needed.
5. Add the bergamot essential oil then beat again.
6. Transfer the body butter to a glass or plastic jar and seal it with a lid.

Sweet Cedarwood Body Butter

Ingredients:

½ cup coconut oil

½ cup cocoa butter

2 tablespoons sweet almond oil

10 drops cedarwood essential oil

Instructions:

1. Heat the cocoa butter in a double boiler over low heat until just melted.
2. Remove from heat and whisk in the coconut oil and sweet almond oil.
3. Let the mixture solidify at room temperature.
4. Whip the body butter on high speed for 5 to 8 minutes, scraping down the sides as needed.
5. Add the cedarwood essential oil then beat again.
6. Transfer the body butter to a glass or plastic jar and seal it with a lid.

Soothing Coconut Oil Body Butter

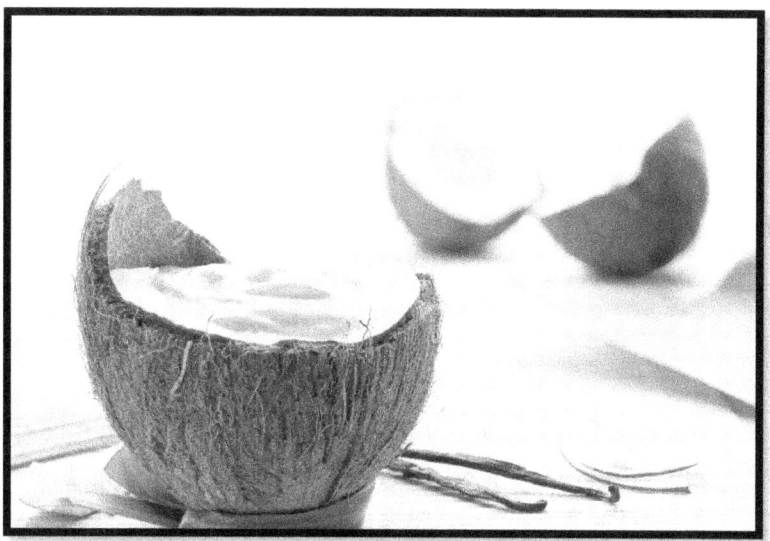

Ingredients:

1 cup coconut oil

1 teaspoon sweet almond oil

2 drops chamomile essential oil

1 drop ylang-ylang essential oil

Instructions:

1. Combine the coconut oil, sweet almond oil and essential oil in a mixing bowl.
2. Whip the body butter on high speed for 5 to 8 minutes, scraping down the sides as needed.
3. Transfer the body butter to a glass or plastic jar and seal it with a lid.

Sandalwood Body Butter

Ingredients:

1 cup coconut oil

1 teaspoon sweet almond oil

5 drops sandalwood essential oil

Instructions:

1. Combine the coconut oil, sweet almond oil and essential oil in a mixing bowl.
2. Whip the body butter on high speed for 5 to 8 minutes, scraping down the sides as needed.
3. Transfer the body butter to a glass or plastic jar and seal it with a lid.

Chamomile Body Butter

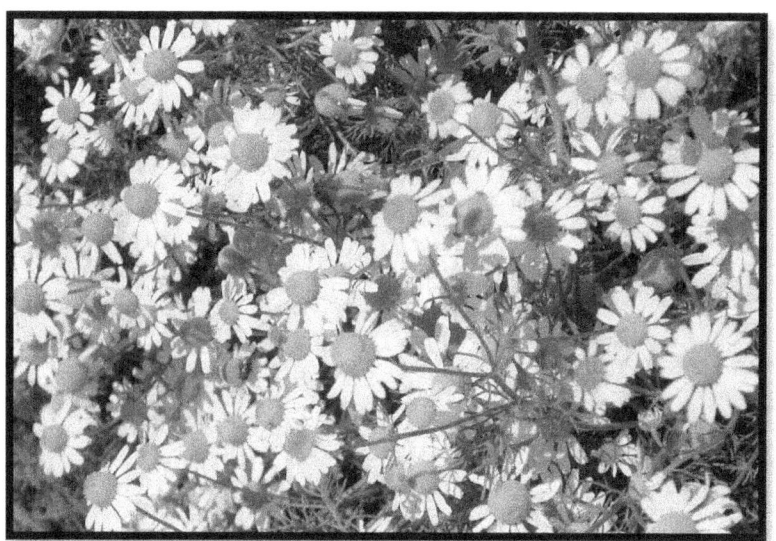

Ingredients:

1 cup cocoa butter

½ cup coconut oil

½ cup jojoba oil

10 to 20 drops chamomile essential oil

Instructions:

1. Heat the cocoa butter in a double boiler over low heat until just melted.
2. Remove from heat and whisk in the coconut oil and jojoba oil.
3. Let the mixture solidify at room temperature.
4. Whip the body butter on high speed for 5 to 8 minutes, scraping down the sides as needed.
5. Add the chamomile essential oil then beat again.
6. Transfer the body butter to a glass or plastic jar and seal it with a lid.

Bug Repellant Body Butter

Ingredients:

½ cup cocoa butter

½ cup shea butter

½ cup coconut oil

½ cup sweet almond oil

10 to 20 drops citronella essential oil

Instructions:

1. Heat the cocoa butter and shea butter in a double boiler over low heat until just melted.
2. Remove from heat and whisk in the coconut oil and sweet almond oil.
3. Let the mixture solidify at room temperature.
4. Whip the body butter on high speed for 5 to 8 minutes, scraping down the sides as needed.
5. Add the chamomile essential oil then beat again.
6. Transfer the body butter to a glass or plastic jar and seal it with a lid.

Mood-Lifting Body Butter

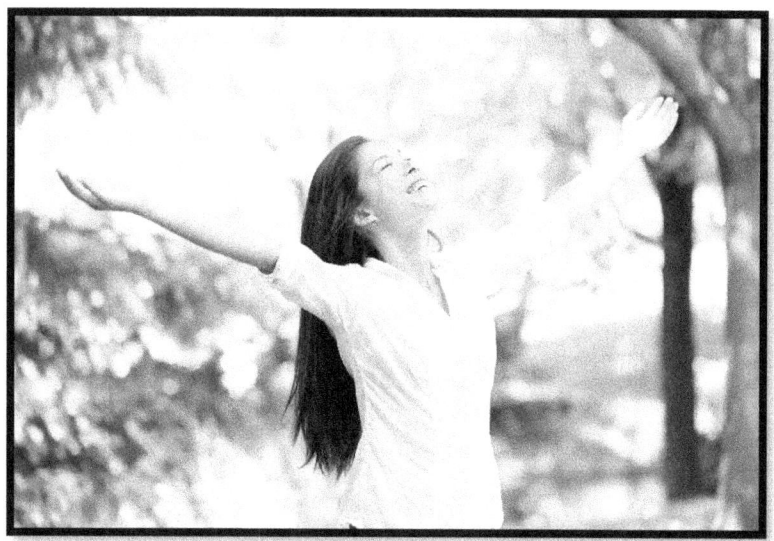

Ingredients:

1 cup shea butter

½ cup coconut oil

½ cup jojoba oil

10 to 20 drops clary sage essential oil

Instructions:

1. Heat the shea butter in a double boiler over low heat until just melted.
2. Remove from heat and whisk in the coconut oil and jojoba oil.
3. Let the mixture solidify at room temperature.
4. Whip the body butter on high speed for 5 to 8 minutes, scraping down the sides as needed.
5. Add the clary sage essential oil then beat again.
6. Transfer the body butter to a glass or plastic jar and seal it with a lid.

Fresh and Floral Body Butter

Ingredients:

½ cup mango butter

½ cup shea butter

½ cup coconut oil

½ cup jojoba oil

5 drops geranium essential oil

5 drops rose essential oil

5 drops jasmine essential oil

Instructions:

1. Heat the mango butter and shea butter in a double boiler over low heat until just melted.
2. Remove from heat and whisk in the coconut oil and jojoba oil.
3. Let the mixture solidify at room temperature.
4. Whip the body butter on high speed for 5 to 8 minutes, scraping down the sides as needed.
5. Add the geranium, rose and jasmine essential oils then beat again.
6. Transfer the body butter to a glass or plastic jar and seal it with a lid.

Jasmine Body Butter

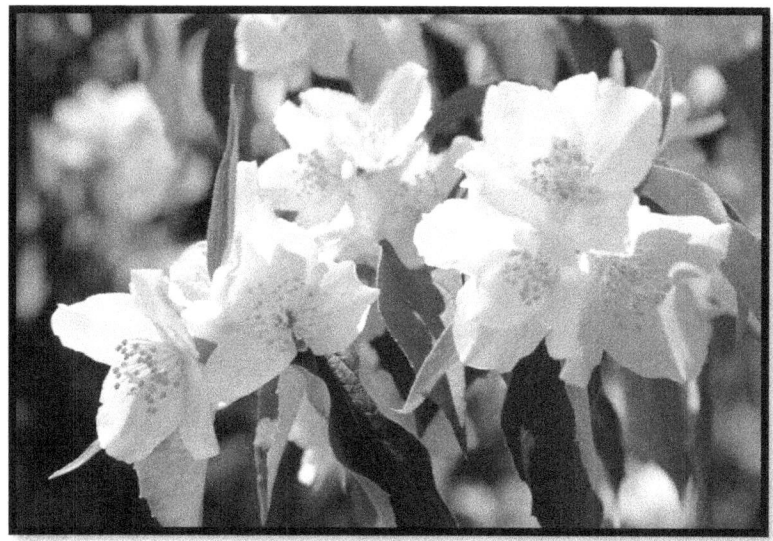

Ingredients:

1 cup shea butter

½ cup coconut oil

½ cup jojoba oil

10 to 20 drops jasmine essential oil

Instructions:

1. Heat the shea butter in a double boiler over low heat until just melted.
2. Remove from heat and whisk in the coconut oil and jojoba oil.
3. Let the mixture solidify at room temperature.
4. Whip the body butter on high speed for 5 to 8 minutes, scraping down the sides as needed.
5. Add the jasmine essential oil then beat again.
6. Transfer the body butter to a glass or plastic jar and seal it with a lid.

Astringent Body Butter

Ingredients:

1 cup coconut oil

1 teaspoon sweet almond oil

5 to 10 drops grapefruit essential oil

Instructions:

1. Heat the coconut oil in a double boiler over low heat until just melted.
2. Remove from heat and whisk in the sweet almond oil.
3. Let the mixture solidify at room temperature.
4. Whip the body butter on high speed for 5 to 8 minutes, scraping down the sides as needed.
5. Add the grapefruit essential oil then beat again.
6. Transfer the body butter to a glass or plastic jar and seal it with a lid.

Lemon Lime Body Butter

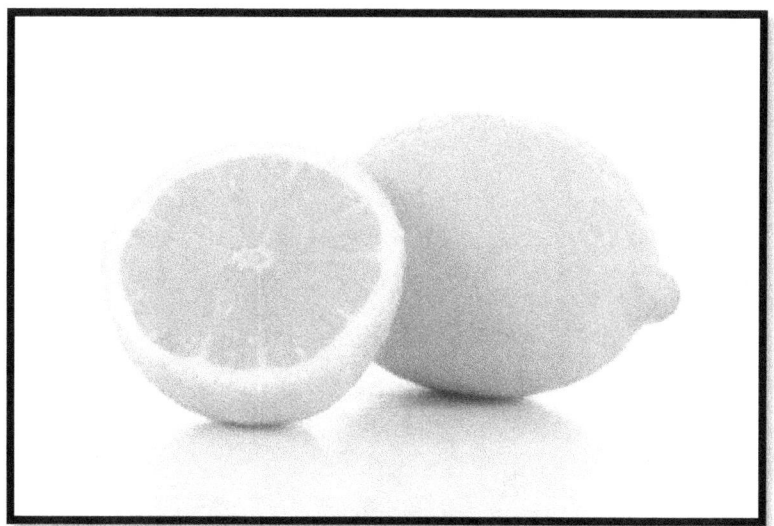

Ingredients:

1 cup cocoa butter

½ cup coconut oil

¼ cup sweet almond oil

1 tablespoon jojoba oil

5 drops lime essential oil

5 drops lemon essential oil

Instructions:

1. Heat the cocoa butter in a double boiler over low heat until just melted.
2. Remove from heat and whisk in the coconut oil, jojoba oil and sweet almond oil.
3. Let the mixture solidify at room temperature.
4. Whip the body butter on high speed for 5 to 8 minutes, scraping down the sides as needed.
5. Add the lemon and lime essential oils then beat again.
6. Transfer the body butter to a glass or plastic jar and seal it with a lid.

www.ingramcontent.com/pod-product-compliance
Lightning Source LLC
Chambersburg PA
CBHW081810280526
45789CB00008B/3078